NEW ASPECTS OF CHEAP FOOD

Printed in Great Britain by Love & Malcomson, Limited, Redhill

NEW ASPECTS
OF
CHEAP FOOD

By

RUDOLPH KELLER (PRAGUE)

D.Sc., BALE

LONDON:

RESEARCH BOOKS LIMITED

in association with

WILLIAM HEINEMANN (MEDICAL BOOKS) LIMITED

1943

CONTENTS

NEW ASPECTS OF CHEAP FOOD

PREFACE

CENTRAL EUROPE, with its poverty and its lack of cheap oceanic transportation, its mountainous districts without sufficient roads and railways, has developed a number of nutritional methods based on the cheapest home-grown foods, in which preference is given to dried curds and sausages and use is made of primitive methods of drying and salting. The mountaineer who has to carry his foreign foods and his tobacco on his back over foot-paths some thousand feet high, learns to economise the small shopping space offered by his shoulders. When one enters his hut one finds only dried herbs, dried sausages, dried curd-cheese, smoked dry meat, dried tobacco, calcined soda, concentrated spirits, and the like. In normal times the Central European eats, as a cheap food, salt herrings—a food of British origin which however is not eaten in Britain itself, because in this country, so near the ocean, fresh herrings are a cheap food. Salt herring and smoked fish represent old methods of preserving fish by withdrawing the water. The modern designation of this process is "dehydration" and this method is now again being used, also in England, to save precious shipping space.

Dehydration is one of the oldest methods for protecting food against putrefaction by microbes, and concentration is another method of reducing the weight and volume of foods and beverages and of making them less accessible to bacterial attacks. Butter-making is another old process for separating the fat from the water in which it is contained in raw milk. Furthermore, the concentration of the albumens of milk in the form of curds and, when dried and ripe, as cheese is another old method of dehydration widely used in France, in the East and in the Alps, where dozens of different varieties of dried curds and cheeses are made. England and Scotland also, particularly the mountainous districts, have their own cheeses which are mostly cheaper than those of the Continent and not inferior to the latter. Another form of concentrated or dehydrated food is roasted bread, or toast, which was first made in the British Isles and has now conquered the whole world under its English name.

The great races of the world have all offered their contributions to cooking and baking processes. The Slav races have prepared a great number of cheap and nourishing dishes, some of which have found their way even to conservative England through Czech and Polish cooks. I am unable to give the recipes of these excellent foods—sausages, vegetables and cakes—some of which cannot be made here, for the reason that the ingredients or the flavourings are not obtainable in England. I can only describe the characteristic differences between Continental and English methods, and try to show that under present circumstances some of the Continental devices might be adopted in order to save a little shipping space.

It is not only shipping space that is short, but also lorry space ; and coal and petrol for local transportation; in addition there is a shortage of man and woman power for shopping, a shortage of bus and tube accommodation for shopping housewives and their helpers, and all these conditions exert a pressure for more concentrated foods or for foods which assemble the vitamins of cooked vegetables either with flour, fats or albumens. These nutritive combinations can already be seen here and there in this country, but they represent the daily nutritional routine in the Middle Eastern and Eastern countries of the world. This is not a plea for the Chinese way of cooking with half-a-dozen unrecognisable ingredients in one dish. I merely wish to emphasize that an approach to the Far Eastern methods by way of the Slav dishes would not only render more palatable some of the poorly cooked vegetables and potatoes, as prepared in this country, but would also be the means of saving some hundred thousand tons of railway truck space and some hundred thousand tons of petrol for lorries, in addition to considerable washing of pots and pans and dishes. The recipes of the Food Ministry appearing in the newspapers often recommend combinations of starchy and vitamin-containing potatoes and vegetables. Following the continental procedures, they herein recommend raw shredded vegetables, which are richer in vitamins and minerals than are cooked vegetables.

The health value of foods is a subject much studied in Central Europe. In my laboratory in Prague many of the colleagues specialised in minerals. I mention in particularly Professor R. Fürth, Physicist of Prague University ; Professor Gicklhorn, biologist at the same University ; Professor Nonnenbruch (Internal Medicine); Doctor Heinrich Waelsch (now in New York) ; Dr. B. Schober (now in London) ; Dr. Luis Nistler, the inventor of a new method of micro-diffusion, used also in America and in England, etc., etc.

Much attention has been given to the subject of mineral diet on the Continent. The leaders of this branch of research were the late Dr. Bircher-Benner, of Zürich ; Dr. Max Gerson, known as " anti-salt Gerson," formerly at the clinic of Sauerbruch in Berlin, now in New York ; Dr. Ragnar Berg, Oslo, Professor Hans Eppinger, Vienna University, as well as his former assistant, Professor Dr. H. Kaunitz, now in New York.

Bircher-Benner, of whose books five have been translated into English, accepted my methods in his lectures. In addition, Eppinger, Kaunitz and Popper have published much work, based on the research of my laboratory at Prague; whilst Ragnar Berg and many others accepted my theory and attributed importance to it. I must also mention that some Americans, such as Edward Singer have elaborated my microscopic methods, whilst Japanese specialists, including Professors Seki and Kuwada, introduced into their country the Prague technique which the latter had studied in my laboratory. In England I am not well known, as Great Britain has no University chairs of Cytology, of Histology and of Biophysics.

I must apologise for quoting my followers in other parts of the world, which however is necessary as I and my co-workers represent a new aspect of biological science which has not yet been fully recognised by Physiological and Pathological Science. Thus far our conception of animal metabolism is familiar only to certain leading physiologists and therapeutists, but not to the general practitioner, who, in Central Europe, for the past sixty years or so has been advocating the low-salt diet but has not been greatly concerned about the theory of mineral diet. Many of the leading personalities in Eastern Europe adopt a low-salt diet, as, for example, Stalin and his eighty-years old mother, whose doctor is my collaborator, Professor Eppinger; so also do Hitler and his entourage acting on the advice of Sauerbruch, the dietitian and pupil of Gerson. I may also cite Professor Salazar, the dictator of Portugal, and many other prominent Continental statesmen. In addition, the patients of the world-famous Lahmann Sanatorium, near Dresden, and of some fifty other sanatoria, are for the most part kept on a diet of uncooked vegetables and low salt, which is potassium-rich and sodium-poor. May I add that I am not an advocate of excessive raw vegetable diets, which systems are followed by some millions of people in Central Europe, including many of the leading politicians. A moderate addition of raw vegetables to one's diet is, however, preferable to cooked vegetables only.

Dr. Gerson was the first person to cure one of the most serious diseases—lupus (tuberculosis of the skin)—by a simple diet of salt-free raw vegetables. Considerable work, attention and patience are needed for initiation into the new aspects and theories of this problem.

After Gerson's expulsion from Sauerbruch's clinics in Berlin, this specialist of modern dietetics came to Britain but found no followers in this country. Gerson is a very modest man, and the English doctors and the public were not prepared to pay attention to this pioneer of modern nutrition. Pioneers have not an easy life in this world, but in England most pioneers have been martyrs. In the British Isles foreign literature is not studied much, and even American literature in the same language is neglected. An insular mentality has developed which has achieved grand discoveries of single geniuses but underestimates the achievements of the Allied Slav peoples and of the enemies. As an example I may quote that a Briton, Professor F. F. Tisdall, of Toronto clinic, has developed the modern methods of microchemical investigation of potassium, sodium and calcium, and that his methods are widely utilised in Germany and in Japan, as well as on the Continent and in America, but Britain is the only country which makes a very modest use of the Tisdall and the Kramer (New York) methods.

It is a pity that men like Bircher-Benner, Berg and Gerson are not so much studied in this country. I do not believe that all results of these reformers are 100 per cent. right and the old ways are 100 per cent. wrong. I am sure, however, that the doctors and the public should look at dietetic problems also from the aspect of those men who have thousands of followers in Central Europe.

VEGETABLES WITH ADDITIONS

ENGLISH dietitians are agreed that vegetables and potatoes constitute a weak point in English cooking. It is a pity that the water in which vegetables and potatoes are cooked is thrown away instead of being utilised for soups and gravies. There is no doubt that vegetables are necessary, very necessary, but when the cooking water is thrown into the sink there remains very little nutritive substance in most vegetables. Moreover, the simple way of boiling greens is primitive also, from the viewpoint of taste and appearance. The physiologist is confronted with a difficult problem when he tries to explain why for centuries past vegetables have been eaten. Science ascribes their beneficial effect to their vitamins, but the vitamin content is not great in boiled vegetables, it is more abundant in fresh, uncooked greens, although even there it is not very high. The nutritive content of starch or protein is mostly only from 1 to 2% : most vegetables consist of 90 or even 95% water, so that the nutritive content, according to present-day methods and knowledge, is very small. It is probable that vegetables, particularly raw vegetables, which for thousands of years have been used by the herb doctors of every race, contain, in addition to vitamins and minerals, some element which is essential for perfect health.

Vegetables can safely be cooked, braised or baked with fat, or they can be eaten raw as salads. Another way is to press the liquid out of them, or to eat them combined with milk, meat, fish or poultry. The French have a preference for vegetables prepared with fat, which makes these dishes very tasty and nourishing ; the Alpine countries in Central Europe prepare potatoes with white curds and call it "Sterz," they add this white cheese also to cakes. In Alpine huts curds and cheese mixtures are the cheapest albumens. Russia and Poland are fond of "borsht," a sort of vegetable soup.

The Slavs eat many greens with a heated mixture of flour and fat. It is similar to English brown sauce. The Czechs mix potatoes with fat, sugar and poppy-seed and call it shkubanky, a very popular dish in Czechoslovakia and nourishing and cheap, but perhaps not suitable for the British palate.

For some time there have been many dried vegetables at moderate prices to be bought at the markets in Great Britain of which some are quite good and retain the flavour. I am told that the housewives do not buy it much, even in winter, when fresh vegetables are scarce. A farmer organisation in Cambridge produces dried potatoes, evaporated at low temperature in vacuum, which contain some of the vitamins and 8% protein instead of 1 or 1½% of fresh potatoes. I should think that the products of the Ministry of Food laboratory in Cambridge under Dr. Barker have a great future even in conservative England.

Some of the leading London catering houses offer to their customers courses of fresh uncooked vegetables at a moderate price. At Lyon's for 6d. or even less one can get raw vegetables in a mixture of lettuce, beet, peas, beans with a little salad cream. I have observed that the thousands of employees in London who represent the majority of the customers of these restaurants greatly prefer for their lunch the usual cup of tea with buns or a slice of cake to the appetising vegetable dishes. Those people are mostly of an unhealthy appearance, although they are the descendants of one of the strongest and finest races in the world. The cause of this may be the bad air of the offices in the City, the life devoid of light and natural pleasures, but in part it is also undoubtedly due to the unwise diet and the love of stimulants.

What is the duty of the housewife in order to avoid these dangers? It is to make the vegetables attractive and to see to it that part of them are eaten fresh and uncooked. The cooking manuals of the late Dr. Bircher-Benner, represented by the Food Education Society of Great Britain, are an excellent guide. The Food Ministry recommended in an advertisement of 8th November, 1942, raw, shredded vegetables for children.

A large proportion of vegetables and potatoes will always be eaten cooked. The continental method, however, of braising or baking them, of adding some fat or albumen to them, or of eating them with fresh milk, cream or cheese, is preferable. Vegetables, particularly cooked and salted vegetables, have very small nutritive value, and it may be that sometimes they do not cover the cost of their assimilation by the body, for the body expends much energy in digesting and absorbing small nutritive percentages of these bulky substances. The Slavs use to shred vegetables which have been cooked with very little water and stir them into brown sauce.

A very tasty addition are peas, both cooked and uncooked. A high-power addition, from the point of view of the dietitian, is that of soya flour or of soyolk, pure or mixed with ordinary flour, which contains also between 11% and 14% of albumen. A flour mixture of three parts wheat (wholemeal) to one part soya contains not less albumen than does meat and a little more than fish. To this mixture is added double its weight of water and one tenth its weight of fat. The experienced cook will find that the percentage of fat is too small, but it is sufficient in the case of soya, which itself has 20% of fat, and very good fat. Other leguminous foods, peas for instance, demand more fat. On the Continent much cabbage and sauerkraut is eaten with potatoes. I have seen many English people who liked these dishes very much, but the majority of the people in this country dislike them.

A dish which is very cheap and nourishing, beside being very tasty, is prepared as follows: carrots are stewed with an eighth of their weight fat and very little water. When they are done a quarter of their weight of soya is added and the mixture boiled for a minute. I eat it without salt, but most English people prefer it with a little salt. Potatoes may also be added to the same mixture. It is very satisfying and one feels no hunger for several hours because the protein is digested slowly and remains at least three or four hours in the stomach.

I believe that in these days, when time is often more precious than money, potatoes and vegetables should not be cooked as separate dishes, except in special cases such as asparagus, the delicate flavour of which is easily spoiled by additions.

Another method of improving the taste and increasing the nutritive value of vegetables is to add bread-crumbs which have been roasted in fat. Continental people eat asparagus, cauliflower and other vegetables, also fresh beans, in a mayonnaise or tartare sauce, or else with bread-crumbs roasted in fat or oil. Bread or toast crumbs roasted in fat are too rich if taken alone, but in combination with vegetables or roast meat they are delicious. Obviously these very dry crumbs which have lost their water content and, as a substitute for water, are soaked in fat often have an albumen percentage of nearly twenty and even higher percentages of fat. They contain also more carbohydrate than other farinacious dishes, as the relative content of starch is also increased by the loss of water. Bread-crumbs are a household waste and may be considered therefore as extraordinarily cheap.

The French bake vegetables with cheese sauce—a method which they call " au gratin." This system of utilising vegetables is both economical and tasty.

At the present time when servants and cooks, in particular, are asking higher wages or are quite unobtainable, the combination of several categories of food on one plate (hot-pots) is advantageous, if only as a labour-saving and fuel-saving device.

COMPARATIVE VALUE OF FOODS

FOODS, as everybody knows, consist of characteristic constituents of different nature. The bulk of them are the energy foods characterised by their caloric values viz., carbohydrates, to which belong the starchy foods (cereals) with some 1,800 calories per lb., fats with some 3,000 calories per lb., and the body-building foods, the proteins or albumens which represent the main constituents of meat, fish, eggs, milk, soya and some legumes. Besides these foods only small quantities of flavouring substances and vitamins are necessary or agreeable, possibly only a small part of 1% of the total intake. Furthermore, there are stimulants like alcohol, thein or caffein, the latter two alkaloids being different names for the same chemical substance ; and in addition there are flavouring substances, most of which satisfy the manifold wants and appetites of mankind. It is not easy to give comparative figures in one denominator to show at a glance the advantages or disadvantages of this or that kind of food. Cattle breeders have a system of evaluation, based on a great number of experiments with cows and pigs. They feed the animals with the different foods and with starchy foods, and designate the comparative value as the " starch-equivalent." Only very few comparative experiments have been made with human beings as experimental subjects, but the cattle foods, so far as men are able to digest them, give us some guidance in this problem.

Another help is given us by the fact that householders of all nations greatly prefer albumens and fats to the starchy foods and pay for proteins fifteen times and for fats four or six times as much as for corn or potatoes. It may be that this estimate is too high if compared with experiments made on animals, but part of it is based on the age-long experience of many races.

We must recognise the fact that both in peace time and in war, people are little interested in their "daily bread," which is available to the poorest family; the prayers of men and women are centred on the desire for more albumen (if we substitute the scientific term for a certain category of food, such as milk, eggs, fish, meat, sausage, poultry), which in the eyes of housewives is the most desirable food. The smallest wages and salaries are sufficient for the daily bread, but not for the "daily protein" or the "daily fat" or the "daily vitamin." These foods make greater inroads on the budget of the poor and of the middle-classes.

This leads us to the attempt to calculate the nutritive contents of foods according to their albumen and fat percentages, with an additional multiplier of five for the albumen and two for the fat percentages. We will take as basis of comparison the potato, which most housewives consider a cheap food, and we will assume that the vitamins, owing to their very small traces (parts of thousandths) quite elude each quantitive estimate. But, as they are as indispensable for nutrition as are potatoes, we will evaluate them as potatoes, in spite of their poor content in nutrients. Thus, for instance, when we compare potatoes with cocoa, with 20% protein and 22% fat, we can say: the cocoa is 144% more valuable than potatoes, together it has 244% of the potato value—100% for its albumen and 44% for its fat content. As cocoa is not too much dearer than potatoes, with 2½-fold nutritive value it constitutes a relatively cheap food. In this connection the fact that the potato contains only 19% of edible starch, only 1% of albumen and not fully 1% of fat, is expressed in the high multiplier. To give another case: refined sugar with 100% carbohydrate is actually cheaper than potato; it has five times more carbohydrate and costs not fully five times more. This, although the sugar price includes the sugar tax, and the potato is subsidised by the Treasury!

Our multiplier is a very rough estimate, it is a compromise between the high evaluation of all peoples and an approach to the starch equivalent of the scientific cattle-breeder. In many cases it is obviously incorrect; for instance in the case of coffee and tea, which are not estimated for their nutritive value but for their stimulative power; but in all cases it gives a comparative value which reveals to the eyes of the simple housewife an important factor in connection with the choice between competing foods. After a glance at the table it will be found that the price is a guide to the quality of a food, but not the only guide. I have no prejudice against potatoes; the English potatoes are excellent; I eat them every day, sometimes twice a day. But I want to emphasise that potatoes, so cheap at the first glance, are partly a luxury food, valuable on account of their content of vitamin C, of which they are the only source for many people during the winter. One can see also that chocolate is not the cheapest food, although with its high content of albumen and fat it is not so expensive as people believe. Very cheap are pulses, so much underestimated in this country; very cheap is cane syrup, disregarded by the Government for human consumption. Soya, rice, flour, bread, biscuits, fish, sausages are relatively cheap foods.

The examination of these comparative values shows

us that, besides the nutritive content, such aspects as palatability, market conditions and the outer appearance influence the prices of foods more than does the content of albumen or of any other substance needed by the body. It is of no use to judge the nutritive value exclusively from scientific considerations, for the age-long experience of so many races who agree in the fundamental evaluation of foods is a fact which should not be ignored by scientists. The whole subject of vitamin research is a matter of only about thirty years; each year brings a new vitamin and nobody knows whether in the favourite foods, in addition to the vitamins, there may not exist some quantitative relationship between their constituents which are so important for the perfect health of the people that the natural foods are preferable in a still higher degree than scientific dietitians are disposed to concede to-day.

My multiplier of protein and fat percentages looks at first sight somewhat complicated, but it is very simple if it be interpreted as an attempt to compromise between the analyses of the foods and the age-long practical experience of many races. The chart indicates some properties of the foods including the observation that the production of animal protein and animal fat costs considerably more than that of vegetable fats and albumens, apart from the fact that the palatibility of the albumen- and fat-rich foods is greater than that of the starchy foods, a rule which does not apply in all cases. It is the first attempt to establish the actual value of foods, and although inaccurate, undoubtedly indicates progress. It should be emphasised that the enemies of democracy have given to this problem years of intense study; that to their householders they have stressed the importance of fat and albumen; that they have begun to synthetise albumens and fats from coal-tar products and from synthetic ammonia. The enemies could be called protein-conscious people, and the

British have also, though with reluctance, elaborated synthetic methods for producing albumens from the nitrogen of the air. The food-content tables in English text books are a little more accurate than the German tables. But the German tables are popular and more intensely propagated.

The figures of the table give no correct indication of the comparative nutritive value of the East Asiatic cheap foods in proportion to their price. They are based on the usual prices in the retail shops, which are high in commodities other than Government-subsidised cereals, which are the staple foods in this country. For instance, the case of soya flour can be quoted, of which an expert in *The Times* wrote as early as April, 1940, that the neglect of this important food is one of the greatest errors of British food politics. The Japanese obtain beans at a price of £8 per ton, corresponding to 1d. per lb., whilst the British who pay high costs for freight and insurance and at least three middle-men, viz., the wholesale, grocery and agency business, pay nearly a shilling, retail, for soya. The manufacturer gets no more than the maximum price, that is 3½d. per lb.; the remaining 7d. represents the cost of distribution. One of the great advantages of soya, its extreme cheapness, is thus lost by this round-about way of distribution not to mention that the cereals and flour are subsidised by the Treasury. Thus, while the enemy eats his staple food at a price of one-half or even one-third of that represented by nutritive units of our potato price, the Englishman has to pay more for this indispensable food.

Another example is treacle, which is so cheap in America and so expensive in Britain. It costs double the price of sugar, because the Government grants molasses only for cattle which, therefore, have record supplies of milk, whilst the human mothers cannot produce enough milk for their children owing to their impoverished physique, due to excessive consumption of refined sugar and other highly processed foods deprived of their natural minerals and vitamins.

The staple food of South-Eastern Europe, maize and polenta, is exceedingly cheap in Rumania and Hungary, and relatively expensive in this country. But even at the high British price cornflour is a cheaper nutrient than potato. During the first years of the war Argentine maize was offered f.o.b. Buenos Aires at £2 per ton, i.e., not fully one farthing per lb.; but it could not be accepted by the British Government, because the public is not prepared to use it and because of formal regulations prohibiting the purchase of commodities from countries which at that time had differences with the Foreign Office, to which group Argentina apparently belonged. Lord Halifax informed the Food Ministry from which countries corn could or could not be purchased.

In spite of all these difficulties it is useful to study these comparative food values. It is obvious that much could be saved in shipping space, in railway space, in lorry space, and in foreign currency if the food problem were handled without prejudice, merely on the basis of the actual value of the nutrient. I am not a fanatic for protein or vitamins, and hold that the palatability of a dish is not less important than its nutritive value; but one may assume that the Eastern nations have also quite good palates, and one should remember that the Chinese are extraordinary gourmets. Thus, with the help of some determination and perseverance an approach to a cheaper method of feeding, based on an observation of the methods furnished by our enemies, seems to be a problem that the poorer world of tomorrow should energetically take up. They can offer us many suggestions as to the solution of this problem, which has not yet received the full attention of dietitians and economists.

It is not permitted from a scientific point of view to add body-building food percentages to energy percentages, such as carbohydrate and fat percentages, but under the assumption that science has not yet discovered all accessory nourishing substances, we may grant some consideration to the practical fact of the general higher evaluation of the albumen and fat, particularly in a time of an albumen, fat and vitamin-blockade and counter-blockade. Another inaccuracy of my table is the fact that many of the foodstuffs are either scarce or unobtainable at the maximum price. But in spite of all inaccuracies the figures are approximately right, as the results are in agreement with the starch-equivalent of the cattle-breeders.

The nutrient percentages are calculated on the base of the figures of Margery Abrahams and Elise M. Widdowson in their excellent book, "Modern Dietary Treatment," 2nd edition, London, 1940. With the aid of this table the reader is able to calculate, for instance, the nutrient value of margarine, containing 88% fat. Margarine has about nine times the caloric value of potato, and, as it costs only 5d., in comparison to 1d., for potatoes, it has a food value of 5-ninths, or 0.55. It is, therefore, much cheaper than potatoes.

The English margarine has a lovely taste, and the Ministry of Food has added the vitamins A and D, the latter the anti-rickets vitamin. It will make disappear rickets, called "English Disease" on the Continent. The growing generation of Britons will have stronger bones and will be 1 or 1½ inches taller than their elders; they owe this to Lord Woolton and to Professor Drummond, who added the vitamins to the margarine. Even the most unfriendly critic of the Food Ministry is obliged to stress this fact, and to recommend the rule of Lord Woolton to eat more potatoes.

EXPLANATION OF THE TABLE

The table is an attempt to give in *one* figure an estimate of the nutritional value of the foods. It is not possible to give an exact figure in the present state of our knowledge of the comparative value of foods. One can give only an approach to the actual value of the single foodstuffs.

The estimate is based on a comparison with potatoes, to-day the staple food of the poorer part of the community and thought to be the cheapest food, which it is not actually. First the nutrient percentages are evaluated with the fivefold value for albumen or protein and with the double value of the fats as an addition to the potato base. Thus a multiplier is obtained which is a compromise between the analytical constituents and between the usual evaluation by the centuries-old experiences of the housewives of the whole world. This method would lead to strange results in the case of fruit and vegetables most of which have neither considerable protein or fat contents, but contain vitamins and minerals which cannot be estimated in percentages. These commodities are, therefore, estimated as equivalent to potatoes which I believe is too low an estimate as the practical experience of the houswives in most countries tend to give them a higher value. Thus the whole table is not exact, only an attempt to bring the culinary wants and appetites in a raw comparison with the results of practical experience and scientific analyses.

The multiplier which gives the relative value of the nutritive content is compared with the price, either with the market price or with the maximum price which gives an equivalent for potatoes. If this equivalent is lower than 1, it is cheaper, if it is higher it is dearer than potatoes. In the case of soya which has a maximum wholesale price this is the base of the comparison.

The cheapness of bread and flour was more striking during the first three years of the war. After September, 1942, the price of bread was raised and the potato price lowered. But bread remains still cheaper.

	Price	% Carbohy.	Protein	Fat	Cal. oz.	Multipl. against potatoes	Price + potato	Equivalent — units
Apples, raw (with skin and core), fresh	–/8	9·8	0.4	Tr.	11	1	10	—
Apricots, dried, raw	1/–	38	5.0	Tr.	56	1	14	—
Arrowroot . . .	—	92	0·4	Tr.	106	5	—	—
Asparagus, boiled .	—	0·7	0·2	Tr.	3	1	12	—
Bacon, middle, smoked	1/11	0·0	4·0	106	115	2·5	12	—
Barley	–/2	72·5	9·0	2	109	5·1	—	**0·9**
Beans, Butter, boiled .	4d.-6d.	17	7·0	Tr.	28	1·3	—	—
Beef, corned . .	—	0·0	23·0	17	66	2·5	—	—
Beefsteak, raw . .	—	0·0	20·0	11	50	2·2	—	—
Beef, topside, roast, lean	1/8	0·0	27·0	11	67	2·5	5	—
Beef, stewed . .	—	0.0	31·0	9	58	2·7	—	—
Beer or ale— (5% alcohol) . .	—	3	0·5	Tr.	18	—	—	—
Beetroot, boiled .	—	10	2	Tr.	14	1	—	—
Biscuits, cream crackers	–/10	58	9	30	164	4·5	3·8	—
Black Currants, raw .	—	7	1	Tr.	9	1	—	—
Black treacle (molasses)	–/8½	68	1	0·0	80	3·5	**1·5**	—
Blancmange . .	—	2	3	4	35	—	—	—
Bovril . . .	—	0·0	30	1	36	2·5	—	—
Bread, Hovis . .	/–4	41	12	4	70	2·7	—	1·5
,, White . .	–/3½	53	7	1	74	2·9	—	**0·9**

Tr. means Trace only.

	Price	% Carbohy.	Protein	Fat	Cal. oz.	Multipl. against potatoes	Price + potato	Equivalent — units
Bread, White, toasted	—	64	10	1	87	4·7	—	0·95
,, wholemeal	–/2½	45	8	2	65	3·2	—	**0·8**
Brussels Sprouts	—	2	25	Tr.	5	1	—	—
Buns, Rock	—	64	6	17	126	5·2	—	—
Butter, fresh	1/7	Tr.	0·3	86	226	1·7	9	—
Cabbage, boiled	–/2	13	21	11	145	2·6	—	0·8
50% soyolk								
Chocolate	2/-	60	6	32	159	4·9	**3·3**	—
Cocoa powder	1/6	35	22	24	126	4·1	**3·4**	—
Carrots	—	1	1	Tr.	2	1	—	—
Carrots with 40% milk substitute	—	—	—	—	—	1·8	**1·8**	—
Currants	—	55	6	15	126	4·2	—	—
Custard powder	–/10	14	3	4	34	2	5	—
Damsons, raw, stones	1/–	9	0·3	Tr.	10	1	—	—
Dates, w. stones	—	55	2	Tr.	56	3	—	—
Doughnuts	—	50	7	16	106	4	14	—
Dripping	1/–	Tr.	Tr.	100	262	3	**4**	—
Dumpling	–/3	24	3	12	61	2·4	—	0·9
Eggs	2/3	—	21	22	82	2·5	**8**	—
Egg Yolk	5/–	—	17	31	99	2·4	18	—
Figs, green, raw	—	10	2	Tr.	13	—	—	—
,, dried, raw	–/5	54	4	Tr.	66	4	**1.2**	—

	Price	*% Carbohy.*	*Protein*	*Fat*	*Cal. oz.*	*Multipl. against potatoes*	*Price + potato*	*Equivalent — units*
Fish cakes . . .	–/9	10	13	14	62	2·7	**3**	—
,, paste . . .	1/–	12	15	10	50	2·9	3	—
Flour, white . .	–/1·5	80	11	1	108	5·5	—	**0·31**
,, wholemeal .	–/1·5	69	12	2	98	5·2	—	**0·33**
Golden Syrup . .	–/9	80	0·3	—	92	5	1·4	—
Greengages, raw .	—	12	1	Tr.	14	—	—	—
Haddock, fresh, fried .	1/2	3	21	9	50	2·2	7·3	—
Hake, steamed . .	—	—	19	3	30	1·9	—	—
Ham, boiled . .	2/6	—	24	14	62	2·3	10	—
Herring, fried . .	1/2	1·5	20	14	59	2·3	5	—
Honey . . .	1/8	75	0·3	Tr.	—	4	6	—
Irish stew . . .	—	7	4	10	42	1·5	—	—
Jam . . .	1/–	70	1	—	81	3·5	—	—
Kidney, sheeps, fried .	1/8	—	28	9	57	2·6	1·9	—
Kipper, baked, w.bones	–/9	—	14	6	31	1·8	4	—
Leeks, boiled . .	—	4	2	—	7	—	—	—
Lemon Juice . .	—	2	0·3	—	2	—	—	—
Lentils, raw . .	–/7	50	20	Tr.	90	2·2	**2·5**	—
Lettuce . . .	—	2	1	Tr.	3	—	—	—
Liver, raw . . .	–/10	2	17	8	42	2	4	—
Lobster, boiled . .	5/–	22	4	—	34	1·7	25	—
Macaroni . . .	–/7·5	75	12	2	108	1·6	4	—
Malted milk, Horlick's .	1/9	75	15	9	102	5·5	3·8	—

	Price	% Carbohy.	Protein	Fat	Cal. oz.	Multipl. against potatoes	Price + potato	Equivalent — units
Margarine	–/5	—	0·3	88	226	2·6	**1·9**	—
Marmalade	–/11	70	Tr.	—	81	3	2·9	—
Marmite	—	—	10	Tr.	12	1·5	18	—
Meat paste	—	4	20	13	61	2·3	6	—
Milk, fresh	–/4·5	4	3	4	19	1·25	3·5	—
Milk, dried	1/6	40	17	30	152	3·3	3·8	—
Milk, condensed	1/–	55	8	12	106	2·6	3·6	—
Milk, with 30% Terramar substitute	–/8½	15	8	4	44	1·5	5·6	—
Milk, skimmed, condensed	–/8	60	10	—	82	2·5	2·6	—
Milk, plus 40 % Watts substitute, 25% water	–/8·5	8	14	4	55	1·8	4·7	—
Molasses	–/0½	82	—	—	110	58	—	**0·4**
Mushrooms, fried	—	2	25	62	—	1·6	6	—
Mustard, powder	—	20	30	30	134	2·1	—	—
Mutton, stewed	1/5	—	24	24	92	2·5	6	—
Nuts, almonds	2/2	9	20	55	170	2·1	10	—
,, walnuts	1/3	5	14	73	156	2·1	6	—
Oatmeal	–/3·5	75	14	8	123	3·8	—	0·8
Quaker Oats, raw	–/3¾	75	14	5	123	3·8	—	0·8
Olive Oil	1/–	—	—	100	264	3	**2·9**	—
Onion, boiled	—	3	1	Tr.	4	—	—	—

	Price	% Carbohy.	Protein	Fat	Cal. oz.	Multipl. against potatoes	Price + potato	Equivalent — units
Ovaltine	—	55	14	8	89	4·8	—	—
Oxo	—	—	30	4	47	2·6	—	—
Pancakes, Flour Ter.	-/8	40	45	15	88	3·5	2·5	—
Pastry, short	—	55	8	30	152	2	2·3	—
Peas, dried, boiled	—	20	7	30	30	1	**2·5**	—
Peanuts	-/8	9	28	50	172	3·4	**2·3**	—
Peaches	—	52	3	Tr.	66	3	—	—
Pears, tinned syrup	—	16	3	Tr.	20	—	—	—
Pineapples in syrup	—	16	3	Tr.	20	—	—	—
Plaice, fried	—	8	19	15	67	2·3	—	—
Plums, dessert	—	9	1	Tr.	11	—	—	—
Plum tart	—	33	2	10	65	3·8	—	—
Pork, loin (roasted)	—	—	20	40	129	2·8	6	—
Porridge, 2½ oz. pt. water	—	8	2	1	14	1·5	—	**0·9**
Potatoes, old	-/1	20	1	Tr.	25	1·0	—	1
Potatoes, old, boiled	—	20	1·5	Tr.	25	1	—	—
,, ,, baked in skins	—	25	2	Tr.	32	1	—	—
,, chips	—	40	4	10	72	3·3	—	—
,, roast	—	25	3	1	38	1·5	—	—
,, new, boiled	—	19	2	Tr.	23	1	—	—
Queen of puddings	—	24	5	10	59	2·7	—	—
Raisins, dried	-/6	65	1	Tr.	76	4	**1·10**	—

	Price	% Carbohy.	Protein	Fat	Cal. oz.	Multipl. against potatoes	Price + potato	Equivalent — units
Rhubarb, stewed	—	1	Tr.	Tr.	1	—	—	—
Rice, polished, raw	–/6	85	5·2	1	112	5·3	—	**0.9**
,, pudding	—	20	5	9	54	2·7	**2·2**	—
Roe, Herring, fried	—	5	24	15	74	2·5	2·8	—
Ryvita	—	80	8	2	106	5·5	—	—
Sago	—	90	0·3	0·3	110	4·5	—	—
Salmon, tinned	—	20	6	6	39	2·1	—	—
Sausage, Beef, fried	—	16	14	19	83	2·1	—	—
Scones, without eggs	—	58	9	14	111	4·75	—	—
Semolina	—	75	12	2	109	5·2	—	**0·95**
Shortbread	—	65	7	28	154	4·2	—	—
Shredded Wheat	—	80	10	3	112	5·6	—	—
Soyolk	—	20	40	20	180	3·4	—	**0·9**
Soya, 25% in wheat	–/2·2	42	20	6·5	150	3·3	—	**0·65**
Sugar, white	–/4·5	100	Tr.	Tr.	116	6	—	**0·7**
,, Demerara	–/4·5	95	Tr.	Tr.	110	5·8	—	**0·8**
Tapioca	—	95	0·3	Tr.	111	5·8	—	—
Tea, as purchased	—	—	15	—	17	1·7	—	—
Tomatoes	—	3	1	Tr.	4	1	—	—
Virol	—	60	5	7	108	4·4	—	—
Vita-Wheat	—	60	10	10	118	4·7	—	—
White sauce, sweet	—	20	3	10	48	—	—	—
Yorkshire pudding	—	24	8	10	65	2·6	2·5	—

THE ECONOMIC SIDE OF CHEAP FOOD

It seems to me that the public underestimates the economic aspect of cheap and scientific feeding. The Lancashire textile worker never fully understood why he lost his job and had to accept unemployment and the dole. This catastrophe had many causes, but one of the chief was that the Oriental worker was fed more cheaply. I am not an advocate of Chinese food for British workers. In spite of everything, I think that the British food, on an average, is better than Chinese or Japanese food. However, Asiatic food is not so much inferior, but very much cheaper, than British food. Japanese food is scientifically on a very high level. Years before the war Japan had great numbers of excellent bio-chemists employed as food supervisors. The Food dictator placed two biochemists in the Imperial palace who were responsible for the meals of the august personage. It was their aim to see that three meals a day should not cost more than 3d. a day. The whole aristocracy and the high financiers were ordered to live according to these principles. Judging by recent reports, however, the cost of living has recently increased in Japan.

Owing to this cheap but good food the Japanese were able to conquer the East Asiatic, some South American and the African markets before they started the war for the military occupation of those countries. I do not think that their example should be followed, but I strongly believe that some of the methods of co-operation existing in Japan between biochemists and economists should be studied and even emulated in the allied countries. Those who admire the obvious evidences of the co-operative planning of battles between the land, sea and air forces see only the superficial aspect. But there exists also a co-operation between the scientific, biochemic and economic authorities in the countries of the enemies which our own organisations have not yet attained. Germany lost the last great war also through the failure of her currency as a result of inflation, and she has learned from this defeat. In collaboration with Japan she has worked hard to make foods which are both cheap and efficient, and it cannot be denied that both countries have made considerable progress in this respect.

At present, since public affairs in Germany and Japan have been put on a scientific basis, no comparative figures are available ; but there is no doubt that conditions have worsened for the Western Powers. This matter has a bearing, not only on military strength, but it is indicative of the general relative standard distribution of civilisation. A worker who is not compelled to use his income merely or mainly for food, can afford more books, more music, a better education for his children, and so forth.

Not only is the private life of the low-wage earner brighter when the price of food does not paralyse all his liberty in spending, but there is a greater volume and a better quality of exportation when food substances are limited to the necessary minimum. We may learn something from the great Slav nations of 230 millions, perhaps destined to be the future governing race in Continental Europe, and whose population can be well nourished on two-thirds of the amount required by the English for living expenses. Such manufacturers as the Czech bootmaker Bata have made their country the leading shoe exporter of Europe, by utilising the most up-to-date technical developments and by supervising the food of their workers, both from the aspect of hygiene and for its cheapness in proportion to its nutritive contents. After all, it is the duty of the authorities, as of the individual household, to eat the most economical foods.

SOLDIERS' FOOD AND WAR

THE Germans boast that they achieved their great victories in the West by the efficient feeding of their motorised divisions with soya preparations. These, they think, are far superior to the English and French methods of catering for the armoured divisions. In Britain the opinion is expressed that the Western army diet is inferior to the German diet. As early as April, 1940, a food expert stated in *The Times* that the unpreparedness of soya reserves was one of the severest defeats of England in this war. I am not in a position to discuss strategical problems, but it seems to me that an army which is not obliged to drag about the large quantities of bulky foods, generally preferred in this country, has far more transport space available for ammunition and other material, essential for the winning of battles. In the *Tribune* of London I read an article by Dr. G. Bourne, who quotes evidence proving that the diet of the English soldier is out of date and practically confined to starch. A member of the R.A.S.C. claims that he was fed on very bad puddings and had rice pudding five times a week—practically an all-starch diet. This complaint sounds very strange to the foreigner, who has the impression that the British eat far more meat than do the Continentals—an inference which is confirmed also by the consumption statistics. That there still exist some antiquated methods of feeding in the British Army may be probable, but some of Dr. Bourne's remarks are perhaps generalisations and all the Services are certainly not fed on starchy foods. The Air Force, for instance, which is one of the most progressive sections of the British Forces, has plenty of soya—the typical high-power protein food—in its diet, and it seems that this diet, copied from the enemy, has been a good choice.

Dr. Bourne also quotes an article from the *New York Journal of State Medicine* by Dr. Gerson, who describes the efforts of the Germans to give their soldiers the most wholesome and efficient food. Stalin also lives on a low-salt diet, as do some European monarchs. Dr. Gerson finds the German army diet very excellent. He was an army doctor in the Great War.

Dr. Bourne thinks, from his experience in the military kitchens, that the soldiers eat too few vegetables because they are badly cooked. He says: " The greens looks like a compost heap in the mess tin," and he concludes his article : " Shall we learn from our enemy, or instead lose all-important battles because we stick to the traditions of roast beef? We must have the fittest soldiers to combat the strains of modern war."

I do not think that the English diet is so terribly bad as Dr. Bourne describes it to be (perhaps, however, with the exception of vegetables), and that the Navy and R.A.F. have won enough battles to prove the contrary; but the standard of nutritional science in Great Britain is not on the same level as other departments of science have attained in the British Isles. Moreover, this undoubted fact perhaps also influences the army diet, as the British, despite the insufficient number of biochemists in this country, do not wish to accept the services of biochemists of foreign citizenship, even when the latter are anti-Nazis by birth or by choice.

Some of my countrymen, the Czechs, who are in the British Forces, are perfectly satisfied with the cooking, although the Czech culinary reputation is very good, and justly so. Nevertheless, Dr. Bourne may be right from a strategical point of view, in stating that the usual starchy dishes with a poor nutrient content may be a hindrance grave to the quick movements which are so decisive in the modern war of armoured vehicles.

MILK

In some countries people have a superstitious love of milk. It is white and appeals to the ladies on account of this attractive colour (so much esteemed at the breakfast table). There is no doubt that milk is one of the few beverages which comes to us in its natural state, and that it is very wholesome for those who eat so much food which has become demineralised and denaturalised by processing, as for example, sugar, flour and starch. Under the circumstances the Government is right to make the greatest sacrifices in order to secure shipping space for evaporated milk from overseas.

Milk, as most natural foods, is very rich in the potassium group, including phosphorus. It is beneficial for public health, in which respect it has few equals. But milk is not just what the layman, or even some experts, think. It is a very weak food and is much diluted by nature for the breast-fed child and the calf. It is a natural food, but natural only for the suckling or the young up to the age of six months. Dr. Goldmann, of the Prague Pediatric Clinic, one of my collaborators, showed at the International Congress of Pediatry, held in Rome in 1937, that young and adult lower animals inhabiting the sea are very rich in the sodium-group and poor in potassium. Adult man, from the point of view of his tissues is also a potassium animal from six months after birth, at which stage he has acquired the normal potassium balance of the adult. Evolution is not only evolution of some special organs, but of the entire chemical metabolism, although this is not visible to the untrained observer. The embryo in its mother's womb is ontogenetically repeating the development of its ancestors, and begins life like its oceanic forebears. Potassium is the characteristic mineral of the higher animals and plants of to-day, even of marine plants and animals.

The case of milk is not as simple as many think. Like table salt, alcohol and other foods, if given in excess, it shows some bad properties. The embryo obtains from its mother a supply of iron in the liver, pancreas, muscles and other organs, with which to meet the small iron-needs of the breast-fed child. But after six months the iron reserves have disappeared and the child becomes anæmic unless given a little fruit juice or molasses. The American pathologists of the Mayo clinic, Whipple and his co-workers, who won the Nobel Prize for their successful studies of anæmia, made their experimental puppies anæmic by feeding them exclusively on milk at an age when other foods are indispensable. Thus, they have proved even an excess of milk to be unsuitable for puppies of an age beyond the suckling stage. It is not only the iron or the copper, manganese or other substances that are deficient, but the natural milk is too watery, as it contains only a maximum of 15% dry substance, to 85% of water—an excellent preparation for an animal which itself has a similar watery constitution. Gradually, however, the water and sodium escape from the tissues, muscles and liver, although adhering to an exclusively milk diet an adult animal with less liquid-need is given a watery milk diet continually.

If the milk diet is already abnormally watery for older children, for adults it very often constitutes a luxury food. I find the so-called milk substitutes with 50% soya and more, a better beverage in many cases than natural milk. Not only are the Orientals, who are very strong, fed with more soya than milk, but even in Europe many people reinforce the milk with various additions, such as suet or flour, or evaporation (yoghurt), or by the addition of sugar, cocoa, molasses, glucose, salt, eggs, lecithine, etc. England also has a number of reinforced milk preparations, such as Horlick's, Benger, Ovaltine, all of which are very good, but perhaps a little expensive. The Swedes whose biochemists are amongst the foremost in the world, add margarine to ordinary sweet and sour milk, and convert it into a delicate nutritious food, which is also very cheap. Swedish children like it and thrive on it, and they look much better than English children of the same class. Strangely enough, the addition of margarine to milk is prohibited in Britain. Presumably it might be considered a sort of adulteration, but adulteration can only be so designated when an addition is surreptitious. A milk which is labelled as including margarine and which moreover is cheaper, much cheaper than the English preparations for reinforcing milk, cannot be instanced as an attempt to deceive the public. The English have a prejudice against sour milk, and the excellent and cheap Yoghurt, prepared by the Express Dairy Company, is not so much used as it deserves to be. There are also on the market very concentrated and palatable medicinal forms of Yoghurt, but these are only sold as a laxative on a doctor's recommendation. In Central Europe fruit-Yoghurt is eaten as a dainty. Two ounces cost twopence or less.

The milk trade in England is in good hands and on an average milk is better here than in other countries with the exception perhaps of Holland and Scandinavia.

It is not prohibited in the private household to add to the milk a flour with 5% extra fat, soya flour or maltmeal, or any other reinforcer which deprives it of the watery taste. It is also permitted to add suet or margarine in order to increase the fat content. The tendency of our age is to eat more concentrated food, which lessens the work of eating. In many foods, such as toast, porridge, biscuits, steaks and chips, the English and Scotch have been the pioneers of the whole world. In the not distant future they will also drink concentrated milk.

High-power reinforcers may be sold only to bakers and food manufacturers, not to grocers and housewives.

They are not used in ordinary housekeeping, as the dough would not rise quickly enough, because the high contents of fat and albumen inhibit the raising of yeast or baking powder. The bakers avoid this disadvantage by beating the dough with sufficient air in centrifuges before adding the raising agent. It is a pity that housewives are not allowed to use these albumen- and fat-rich reinforcers for cakes, sausages sauces, porridge and soups during the shortage in fats.

The good sorts of milk-substitutes are only a shade cheaper than milk, but much more nourishing. They should be called not substitutes, but ration-extenders.

GENERAL RULES

How should we arrange the four classes of main nutrients in order to secure a substantial diet with given rations and income?

The leading group, the flours and potatoes, constitute the bulk of the unrationed foods, and of the present diet, of which mainly two carbohydrates, sugar and treacle, are at present rationed. No housekeeper needs advice on this subject; all of them use as much as possible of these carbohydrates. I repeat that the cheapness of potatoes is generally over-estimated, on account of its four-fifths water content and its very low content of protein and fat. But it contains enough vitamin C, if one eats half a pound a day, and its delicate albumen gives it a fine taste. The housewife does not know that the flours also belong to the substances richest in albumen; with the exception of rice, which is the poorest in protein, oatmeal, barley, rye, corn and particularly wheat, contain between 11 and 13% protein; Hungarian wheat and some varieties of Canadian wheat contain not less than 13·7, some wholemeals even 14% albumen. This is the reason why mixtures containing eggs, milk,

milk powder, cheese, meat are so very nourishing; mixtures containing pulses, particularly with soya bean, easily raise the albumen content to 18% (the content of fish), the albumen content of other pulses raises it to above 20% (protein content of meat). With much soya albumen contents of 30% and more may be obtained—a record which can be attained by no other addition.

The second important nutrient is albumen or protein, of which animal protein is much preferred for human consumption, on account of its palatability, digestibility and flavour. Proteins are controlled and rationed in all the countries at war. Only fish, certain sausages and the internal organs (offal), such as liver or kidneys, are not rationed; but these are rather scarce. Even in peace times the albumens are the chief concern of the housewife, and they are of paramount importance in war times. There is a wide range of difference in the prices of albumens of animal extraction.

The protein of cheap fish costs a few pence per lb., and the protein of caviar or of lobster between 50 and several hundred shillings per lb. The amount and quality of the albumen the housewife can afford depend on her budget.

The third important nutrient is fat, which is a fuel rather than a body builder. In the latter capacity it is only utilised by adipose persons, but it is also necessary on account of the vitamins which it distributes and of the fat-soluble vitamins A, D, E, F and K, which are carried by the fat through the walls of the intestinal tract. Continental observers have shown that in the absence of fat, or with the addition of vaseline as a laxative, many of the fat-soluble vitamins leave the body unutilised. It is probable that additional so far undiscovered properties of the fats make them indispensable for a normal diet.

There remains the third important item of nutrition,

viz., the vitamins. Here I may be brief, as England has long been the home of the vitamins, and we owe to this country many important experiments and studies on the vitamin question. Of recent years the leading authorities on the vitamin questions have been the Americans, and very much has also been investigated and discovered about vitamins in comparatively small countries, such as Sweden, Holland, also in Japan and the Argentine. In some special fields the European continent now takes the lead and the Slav and even the German biochemists are more aware of the limitations of our present knowledge of the known vitamins, and they take into account the unknown, hitherto, unidentified vitamins by insisting on meals consisting in part of uncooked food and salads, which they assume to contain some unknown "accessory foodstuffs." This unknown element was the original designation of "vitamins" by their first discoverer, Hopkins.

Another important constituent in a complete diet is represented by the minerals, highly valued in Japan and Germany but undervalued in England. The minerals, such as iron, calcium, copper, manganese and cobalt, which are necessary in very small quantities, are called "mineral vitamins" on the Continent—a happy designation—of the minute particles or traces which exert such a profound influence on the equilibrium of nutrition. It has long been known that iron deficiency in the diet leads to very serious illness and even to death. No more than 8 milligrams of iron and half a milligram of copper, according to English investigators, and still less, according to American authors, suffices to cure anæmia caused by lack o f iron.

Endeavouring now to formulate some general rules for a completely palatable and not too expensive form of nutrition, we would say that the point of greatest importance is the substitution of a portion of the not only dear, but partly unobtainable animal protein by vegetable albumen. I have never been a vegetarian and eat nearly my full ration of meat, milk, cheese and egg, even in war-time. But I hold that nobody should try to eat more protein, for the reason that the importation of meat and of cattle-food constitutes a heavy burden on shipping and costs the lives of so many seamen and airmen to whom we are so greatly indebted. To them we owe our continued existence and no one should lay so heavy a burden upon their broad shoulders as we are doing by the consumption of more than our liberal meat rations. Most Continental observers, including myself, are of the opinion that an excessive consumption of meat impairs the health of the average man.

Thus the first rule to be adopted is to restrict meat and egg consumption in favour of more potatoes and bread. The Slavs and Germans mix the albuminous foods with potatoes and vegetables and add bread, rye bread in the East, wheat in the West, and maize in the South. One has to bear in mind that the dry substance of bread, dumplings, puddings and porridge contains some 11 or 12% of protein alone, or about 60% of the albumen content of meat.

The second rule is the utilisation of the cooking water with its rich content of vitamins and minerals for gravies and soups. The Ministry of Food implores the housewife to preserve the water in which potatoes and vegetables have been cooked ; the French and the Slavs do this, but the people of Great Britain obstinately persist in throwing down the sink these valuable food materials. This is particularly regrettable in view of fact that the Germans control 68% of the potassium of the world and are trying to starve the allied nations out of potash, which is the main constituent of the water in which animal or vegetable food has been cooked. The Germans have specialised in research into the qualities of potash and have definitely established that the highly processed foods are deficient in potash and allied substances. It is possible that they hold a rather exaggerated view, but on the other hand, the English opinion that we consume sufficient potassium is a grave error.

The third general rule is that England should follow the example of most of the other nations by starting to adopt the soya bean as a nutrient of albumen and fat. This should be done in connection with the preparation of vegetables (one of the weakest points in English cooking, by which the vegetables are deprived of the most valuable vitamins and minerals). The French prefer to bake or roast their vegetables in fat, the Central Europeans mix potatoes and vegetables with curds, which is very cheap. Both methods are good but not practicable at the present time, as curds are not popular as a dish in this country and fats are strictly rationed during the U-boat blockade. The writer braises his vegetables, potatoes, leeks, etc., with soya and very little suet, margarine and equal parts of water and soya containing 20% of fat, sometimes with peanut with 51% fat. This is not only a very nourishing, but also a very tasty dish. It is served in casserole and whenever tried by the uninitiated this combination of food is highly praised, and the good opinion is reinforced by the significant fact that the guests can never have enough of it.

The discovery of the soya bean by the English public will mark a new epoch comparable to that of the discovery of white flour or of the potato.

Another important reform should be that part of the refined sugar should be substituted by cane syrup. But this reform cannot be carried out by the public as long as the Ministry of Food refuses to grant permits for the importation of cane syrup. Hitherto this molasses has been reserved for cattle consumption, although some of the cane molasses is better than refined sugar and also more wholesome. The fact that the factory price of molasses is about £6 per ton and that of refined sugar £20 per ton, without the tax, indicates that millions of pounds would be saved on foreign purchase; moreover the mothers themselves would be healthier and would produce more and better milk for their children. At present cows in England enjoy much better health than do women, and calves better health than children. But I repeat that only a part of the sugar consumption, not the whole, should be substituted by molasses.

SWEETENING

CARBOHYDRATES are obtainable in abundance in peace and war time, with one exception, viz., sugar. The housewife has to economise sugar, two-thirds of which are imported from abroad during peace time. Formerly, raw cane sugar was a staple food in England, but now Demerara and other brown cane sugar can only be obtained with the greatest difficulty in London. The same over-estimation of the white colour and outer appearance has led to the over-consumption of white flour, often artificially bleached. The English are bound by the same love of the white colour, as a sign of purity, that has dominated the housekeepers of all climes and increased the demand for the highly processed and artificially refined sugar. England has the record consumption in Europe of refined sugar, as the average person of the higher income classes eats no less than 2lbs. a week.

American dietitians had for some time past suspected that white flour and refined sugar are two of the main causes of anæmia and dental decay. The Massachusetts High School of Technical Science in Boston made a systematic investigation of the sweetening problem, as a result of which it was found that the American communities which consumed only refined sugar were not so healthy as the communities which were in the habit either of eating molasses (in the Southern States of the Union), or of chewing raw cane. Later, other investigators tested the molasses diet, and came to the same conclusion as the Boston investigators. It was found that molasses contains more assimilable iron and other minerals than spinach, besides which it appeals to the children's palate.

Investigations showed that England and Scotland had industrial districts in which 73% of the women and 45% of the children were anæmic. Doubtless this was not entirely caused by refined sugar, but I believe that the immoderate consumption of highly processed sugar contributes to this deplorable state of health. The Government refuses to allow the importation of cane molasses, except for cattle. Occasionally, some black treacle (which is cane molasses) is obtainable ; but granulated sugar is most generally consumed. Whereas the Governments of the enemy countries encourage the use of saccharine and dulcin for sweetening purposes, the Food Ministry of Great Britain demands that only a small amount of such sweetening stuff be consumed.

Molasses, a waste product of sugar manufacture is much cheaper than sugar itself. Cane molasses is palatable, but the same does not apply to molasses produced from the beet. Molasses costs £6 per ton, and the maximum price in England was just over a ½d. a lb. without the sugar tax which is about the same amount. Thus, although the total would be very cheap for the poorer classes, it is not on account of its cheapness that I advocate the use of molasses, but for its dietary value for women and children. The finest grade is the cane molasses from the Dutch East Indies. The Dutch are very excellent chemists, and particularly good biochemists. This small nation has won per head of its inhabitants, more Nobel Prizes for Natural Science than any other country.

For sweetening purposes the Germans use a mixture of two-thirds saccharine and one-third dulcin, which they assert is sweeter and better tasting than pure saccharine.

Artificial sweetening is spoiled to some extent by long cooking or baking. It is more efficacious when added at a later stage of the preparation, during cooling, or in the form of liquid syrup or jam. Contained in solid powders or in baked dry cakes it is disappointing, owing to its very slow solubility. As it takes a few minutes to reach the taste nerves, this artificial sweetening often produces only an unpleasant after-taste, when the food has already left the mouth. Not many bakers are able to choose the right quantity that should be used.

Sweetening is not always a matter of content or of substance, but it is important to aim at the nerve end plates in the mouth and to make the sweetness easily accessible to these nerves. An intelligent housewife is able to do much sweetening either with sugar or with synthetic chemicals when she learns to aim at the taste nerves.

BEVERAGES

The first qualities of liquors in the world are mostly of Anglo-Saxon origin. When a dealer in alcoholic drinks in Near Eastern countries wants to boast of his best bottles he always says that the whisky is genuine Scotch whisky, the gin English gin, the porter or stout from London. On the Far Eastern side of the globe American drinks with New York names have a great market. When I was in Scandinavia for a few months I expected to find Swedish punch on the tables ; but, being too sweet, however, it is not much drunk as a regular beverage. In Swedish houses whisky is the leading alcoholic beverage, as in most other European countries.

English porter beer is much admired by connoisseurs on the Continent, but is not much drunk. It cannot be imitated abroad. The beer which is chiefly imitated in Central Europe and in America is the Bohemian Pilsener beer. Only very rarely, however, does it attain the genuine Pilsener, which in the times preceding the blockade was a great export commodity of Czechoslovakia. The Czech breweries have plenty of other beers of weak alcohol percentages which are more characteristic of the skilled work of the excellent Czech workers, of which all Czech manufacturers of foods, sugar and confectionery profited. There are beers in Czechoslovakia the qualities of which in proportion to the price are much more astonishing ; for instance, the beer of Smichov, a suburb of Prague. The Smichov brewery sells more beer than all the three world-famous Pilsen breweries combined. It costs 2d. a pint, and not a barrel is exported but all these 900,000 hectolitres go down Czech throats. I believe that in the not too distant future the new English beers will perhaps be weaker in alcohol content, like the Smichov type, and that they will be drunk at a lower temperature, which is more suitable for weak beers. The beer tax in this country is so high at present that an attempt to make the beer cheaper by less alcohol would here also be very successful. Such a low-grade beer cannot be drunk as warm as the British are accustomed to take it ; but refrigerators are very inexpensive nowadays, much cheaper than the high tax, and with a little more extract-substance the beer tastes very good and is not so heavy in its effects on metabolism. The brewers in England make very good beer, the Whitbread, Barclay and some other brands being excellent. In general, the English beer is an honest beer.

The brewers of the whole world, including the British, blame themselves excessively ; they are strongly influenced by the exaggerations of the popular anti-alcohol movement, more so than the drinkers of their beer. Many of them esteem themselves to be poisoners of the people. In this they are wrong. It is a mistake to consider beer a mere alcoholic drink. Under given circumstances beer or tea or any other plant-extracts are a necessity of ordinary diet on account of their mineral vitamins and other substances lacking in the usual diet. I maintain, and many observers on the Continent are of the same opinion, that a man who is overfed by sodium-chloride (table salt) and underfed in the natural minerals of plants, needs some plant extracts, be they the tea plant or the coffee shrub, or barley or hops, to compensate for the staple foods, such as over-cooked potatoes and vegetables, refined sugar and the like, which are deprived of their valuable contents of phosphorus, potassium, iron, copper ; whereas beer, tea and coffee or cocoa contain a great number of indispensable minerals and perhaps, in addition to the known vitamins, others hitherto undiscovered or not yet identified.

The Englishman likes to find in his food and drink a substantial amount of albumen, or fat or alcohol or strong alkaloids, such as caffeine. Thus, most of his beverages are full of substance and are sometimes too rich. The light beers of the Continent, which are not exportable on account of the large water content, the light wines of France, Austria and Hungary, which are not worth the freight costs and are nearly unknown in England, are sometimes more tasty than the heavy British beverages. Moreover, they are cheaper, not only in production costs, but in taxes, which are the main components of the selling price. The English lose some of the most agreeable beverages because tax and tradition compel them to drink heavy beers and wines when weaker beverages would be more wholesome for them. It is a pity that these delicious drinks which please English travellers so much are excluded from the market, and that the poorer classes never drink a light wine—one of the best things in life. I am sure that the brewer who will be the first to offer the English public a good but mild beer or wine will do a good service to the people, besides making a fortune.

There is another beverage which is neglected here because it is cheap and easily obtainable, viz., cocoa. The public queued before the chocolate shops when the 2d. bars had arrived, but nobody cares for the cocoa which is offered in good qualities and is comparatively cheap. It can be converted into chocolate by the addition during cooking of sugar or saccharine, or better still, a mixture of ¾ saccharine and ¼ dulcin, with a little cooking fat and a trace of vanillin. What is called the chocolate-taste is mostly the scent of the vanillin, which in America and on the Continent is flavoured by a little coumarine and ethyl-vanillin. Cocoa pure and in combination with milk is drunk very much on the Continent. It is one of the most powerful natural nutrients, being very rich in indispensable minerals and very tasty with or without the addition of flavourings such as vanillin. Some people do not like cocoa because they believe it is constipating. This is not the case, but whoever thinks it is may add a little magnesium carbonate, thereby converting it into a mild laxative.

Cocoa prepared with a little saccharine or sugar is also a refreshing summer drink, and if preferred, vanillin flavouring may be added.

The English beverages are very good, but rather dear. The cheap drinks are affected by the general suggestion that what is cheap is bad. This may be true in some cases but not in all. The Continent consumes cheaper beverages which are not always worse, but sometimes even better.

SALT AND POTASSIUM

(*This chapter is for Scientists only*)

OUR Prague group of investigators has often been called the "electrostatic" school, because some 120 of our 200 papers dealt with the localisation and the measurements of the electric charges of living microscopic cells, to which we ascribe a certain importance in cell physiology. After giving a series of lectures at the University of Basle in Switzerland, at which some thirty professors and about eighty younger followers from several countries of Central Europe attended as listeners, we won the interest and collaboration of some of the leading medical authorities, as, for instance, Professors Spiro and Dr. Jösta Ekehorn, Professor Eppinger and his assistant Professor Kaunitz ; Dr. Edward Singer, New York; Roller and Schober, Professor Nonnenbruch and Professor T. G. Mueller, Professor O. Klein and Dr. Heinr. Waelsch. Many other pathologists and therapeutists found that our methods and results could be tested in connection with medical and dietetic problems. Ellinger and Hirt, Karl Spiro, Kaunitz and Eppinger improved on many of our methods and have adapted them to medical problems. Subsequently, other practitioners, including Professor Nonnenbruch and Professor Epstein, as well as a number of dietitians, became interested in our methods. After the death of our friend Spiro other biochemists of international reputation, such as Professor Abderhalden and Professor Carl Neuberg, became familiar with the new microbiophysics, and in Abderhalden's Institute, Professor Wertheimer elaborated many units of the contrasting electric groups and elucidated problems hitherto deemed insoluble. Professor Fodor, another former assistant of Abderhalden, wrote a book on Microphysiology in which he introduced the Prague methods and theories.

With the help of our micro-electrodes Kaunitz has measured the cell electricity of animals in a normal state and after poisoning. He found the electric forces of pathological cells in general lower than those of normal cells. He was able to show, with the methods of F. P. Fischer and Ellinger, that such diseased cells do not possess the repelling force of electro-positivity, and that the table salt enters the muscle, heart and liver cells, where it acts as a weak poison. When Professor Eppinger was chosen to deliver the festival lecture on the occasion of the four hundred year Anniversary of Vienna University 1936, he chose to demonstrate the microphotographs of Roller and Schober, showing the entrance of the electro-positive group, salt and water, into the electro-positive tissues where they are noxious. This phenomenon is called "œdema" in scientific medicine and it cannot be understood without some knowledge of the distribution of the electric forces in microscopic cells. All investigators who have studied these facts believe that in the near future the knowledge of the electric power-centres of the living cells will be as necessary for a doctor as the knowledge of topographic anatomy.

The fact that two antagonistic groups are wandering in contrary directions from each other could not remain undiscovered. Under the name of "intracellular" and "extracellular" groups they are well known and have been investigated in America. This designation is partly right, partly inaccurate. There are many sorts of cells, the bile capillaries of the liver, the male sex-cells, the parietal cells of the stomach, which are electro-negative, sodium-rich and potassium-poor within the cells, and for which the designation "intra"-cellular for potassium phosphate is, therefore, wrong. In the vegetable kingdom the assimilating cells are negative and the juices positive. They have, therefore, the potassium groups outside and the sodium group inside the protoplasm.

The Slav nations have made many practical experiments on salt. The Russians unknowingly made a great mass experiment during the first World War. The food conditions in Leningrad were so bad that the population lived a long time on salt herrings from the nearby Baltic Sea. They were stricken with many diseases, and the horrible disease of eclampsia, an œdema of the pregnant woman, was very widespread. On the Eastern side of the great Empire, in Kasan, a salt famine broke out, owing to the miserable transportation conditions. Kasan enjoyed an excellent state of health, with very few cases of eclampsia.

To return to the practical question of salt over-feeding, to the consideration of which problem the collaboration of some dietitians has led us, it should be said that the practical results are independent of the question whether salt in living cells is electro-positive or not. It will be more easily understood if I give some facts of how our groups of scientists, joined the anti-salt reformers, one of whom, Gerson, visited me in Prague and studied our methods. The discovery of œdema as an electric disturbance with an excess of sodium in muscle and liver suggested the advisability of being very careful in giving table-salt to patients, and some medical friends of great experience supported this conclusion. Thus, our medical collaborators tried out on some patients the whole potassium group, which had been termed "Equilibrin." The treatment proved to be quite successful in many cases and without effect in other cases. The most surprising thing was to note the powerful effect produced in many skin diseases, on which Dr. Erwin Pulay, Vienna, has first directed my attention. Although my knowledge of medicine or Dermatology was very slight, it was soon obvious that we had discovered some progressive principle. One of the first reports came from a colleague of our laboratory, a doctor of Franzensbad, Erwin Spiegl—now in Boston—who wrote that he had cured hay fever, allergy and asthma by the use of potassium group. About that time I received a letter from Professor Jan Tregr, head of the Dermatological Clinic of Bratislava (Pressburg) University. He said that he had administered the potassium group to gonorrhœa patients and had observed a shortening of the period of cure from five to seven days. We wrote him a polite letter of thanks, but could not believe so unexpected a result. Without any experience of this skin affection it seemed obvious to me that this investigator was exaggerating. Then I forgot about Tregr until some time later when he sent a confirmation by the Prague Clinic of Dermatology to the effect that Tregr's report had been examined and found correct. At the same time Dr. Jacobsohn, a Paris dermatologist, had administered Equilibrin to patients afflicted with gonorrhœa at the dermatological hospital of the Sorbonne, without knowing anything about Tregr, and he in his turn obtained the same results. At that time Dr. Pulay wrote that 25% of his excemas showed a striking improvement after a potassium diet. Dr. Pokorny healed hay fever with Equilibrin, and other favourable reports came in from various quarters. It was obvious that allergic skin affections were often caused by too much of the sodium group. Dr. Pulay was an authority on the effect of diet on skin diseases.

Meanwhile Tregr was extending his experiments to his own department of Lupus. He had some fifty or sixty patients each year suffering from this form of tuberculosis of the skin, which had first been healed by Gerson. For the female department Tregr prescribed the Gerson diet and local treatment, with additions of the potassium group. Soon the improvement of the women patients was so far ahead of the male controls that the men, many of whom were relatives or friends from the same villages in Slovakia, revolted and demanded the same medicine. It was accordingly given to them as well, and the result being the same, the success of this method was proved.

Soon we had plenty of other reports confirming the results of Prague and Bratislava. Pulay in Vienna combined the potash-group treatment with doses of vitamin B and C and with other methods of treatment. The best-known Prague specialist in Internal Medicine, Professor Otto Klein, now in the Argentine, once said to me that, according to his estimate, not less than 40% of his patients were either underfed in the potassium group or overfed in the sodium group. Subsequently I found in Lahmann's publications, and still more distinctly in Bircher-Benner's books and in Gerson's papers that they had all deprived their patients of salt and given them potassium in the form of raw vegetables, salads and fruit juices. This they did until 1937, merely on the assumption that Nature had provided the natural foods for mankind and that we cannot remain healthy without a certain percentage of fresh and undevitamised foods.

All these authors describe how eczema and a few pustules, which disfigure so many faces, disappear after a few raw vegetables and some low-salt diet. I had many experiences of this fact with my potassium group.

Central Europe and other parts of the world have already produced scientists and physicians who are convinced that microphysics and micro-chemistry, particularly the investigation of the small electric forces of the living cell, represent the key to many problems of pathology and therapeutics, for the reason that the minute forces of the living cell grow in inverse ratio to the distance of the two electro-statically charged bodies. According to Coulomb's square-law this equals a thousand-fold field-strength compared to the distances of whole centimetres in the dimensions of the naked eye. The laws of Cavendish and Coulomb make the electro-static force of attraction and repulsion one of the leading forces of the cell. We believe that our body cells are microscopically small, chiefly on account of the electro-static force which is able to act efficiently only over extremely short distances. This sounds strange to persons who possess only a non-microscopic mentality and who are unacquainted with the physics of minimal distances, under which conditions such forces are very powerful. We believe that within a few years the physics of the microscopic cell will develop into a science similar to the physics of the atomic and sub-atomic distances in which electro-static attraction and repulsion is much stronger even than in living cells, because the distances are a million times smaller.

This may seem paradoxical now, but in a few years' time it will be a well-known and commonplace fact that an electric charge of some twenty millivolts influences our diet and nutrition ; that it decisively influences our good and bad health, and that it is positively injurious for us to eat an unbalanced diet, whether this be too electro-positive or too electro-negative.

The paradoxical fact to which our laboratory has dedicated so much time and some 6,000 analyses, viz., that potassium, considered by inorganic physical chemistry to be the most highly electropositive element, apart from rubidium, is adsorbed by negative corpuscles, owing to its strong positivity, and that moreover it wanders to the positive electrode, in the presence of an excess of protoplasmic colloids (first observed by Russian bio-chemists and later studied quantitatively by Waelsch and Kittel in Prague) is of great practical importance, the full understanding of which necessitates some familiarity with the subject. A Rumanian expert, Dr. Urbeanu, who was Food Dictator of the Rumanian army in the first World War, assumed, with some exaggeration, that the

Western Powers lost many of their first battles through their ignorance of the potassium problem. The English do not pay much attention to the fact that a large content of potassium is evidence of a large content of many other indispensable minerals and vitamins which are mostly charged negatively under biological surroundings.

Most biochemists who analyse foods think one or two grammes of potash is enough for the average consumer. This would be correct under natural conditions, but not with our present diet which contains so many denaturalised, demineralised, highly processed and refined foods, as well as an excess of some 15 or 20 grammes of sodium and chloride daily, in the average diet. Apart from the properties of the potassium itself, this is an indicator of the contents of other indispensable accessory foodstuffs, such as lecithin, iron, copper. The Chinese showed great practical wisdom in realising that the soya bean was extremely nourishing. They never knew that soya possesses the record content of potassium, viz., 1½ per cent. The same intelligence was shown by the ancient Aztecs of Mexico when they invented chocolate, and by Americans by their consumption of peanuts.

Germany at the outset of the war initiated a most successful blockade of potash of which the British public to this day is blissfully ignorant; in other words, the German Government made it impossible for us to obtain German potassium. The British Ministry of Health advised the doctors to prescribe sodium instead of potassium compounds. For 42 years, since Loeb received the Nobel prize for it, the world knows that in biology and medicine the sodium acts as an antagonist of potassium.

Printed in Dunstable, United Kingdom

91221475R00030